Longevity ZEN

Roditch Roditch

Contents

Introduction

A see-saw best describes how to look at longevity. You are either up with your health and down with disease or vice versa, and right now, are you going up or down with your health? This small book will look at obvious things like diet and exercise, but it will also look at spirituality, meditation, love, happiness, and community life. Stress, glyphosate in your food, contaminated water, and air are all knocking your health "off balance." Organic food, pure water, fresh air, relaxing exercise, and a joyful spiritual life are taking you "up."

For years, I have wondered how supermarkets can legally sell food contaminated with cancer-causing chemicals that lack basic integrity. Mike Adams, the "Health Ranger," is doing scientific testing of supermarket food and has discovered the obvious truth: poisonous chemicals are in the plant, and yes, your children are eating cancer-causing breakfast cereals every day because you have bought them. The rain does not wash away poison, and washing your food (if you can) does not get rid of the poison. Your food, your water, and the air you breathe are saturated with chemicals that are killing you. Ok, so that's the first step in longevity: only eat organic food, organic air, and organic water, and never shop in a supermarket again; they don't deserve your money or support; they are knowingly killing you for profit.

The issues in this book, in the end, are easy to understand. Live a healthy life in every way, and you will probably have a long one. The psychology of why we don't is beyond me, but I can think of a few reasons why we don't love ourselves enough to be healthy and strong: you never grew up, and so you don't take responsibility for your life. You trust everyone to do the right thing with your health. You are addicted to sugar and salt. You are putting it off until tomorrow because you don't have time to think right now. You have no self-discipline. You like all this junk, including alcohol, because it "temporarily" makes you feel good. It's not the American way to eat healthy food—give me a T-bone steak.

No matter the psychology of why you are not healthy, how about accepting the clear fact: if you don't have a well-balanced healthy lifestyle, you will die before your time. There are so many benefits of a healthy lifestyle apart from living a long time: more energy, fewer visits to the doctor, a closer connection to nature, huge savings on food and health bills, and feeling more positive and in control of your own life.

I have witnessed the passing of friends and family members—not a happy time for anyone and usually well before their time. My mother because of smoking; my father because of a poor diagnosis by his doctor; and friends who had no access to CBD oil Doctors lack the intent and the means to cure you once you fall ill. They are so busy "spending their money" that they do not give you enough time to look at all the options properly. They are also (this is changing) against herbs and nature-based cures. Because we don't take responsibility for our health, we run to the doctor frequently with ailments that can be easily cured at home. This dependence on people who have limited powers to help you is a big problem, and the only way to fix this problem is to accept that doctors are not healers; they are drug facilitators (whether the drugs work or not). Once you understand this, you can gradually build your knowledge to help your body heal itself.

Air

Air is the most important substance for our long-term health. We need to breathe a lot of it every day, and it needs to be pure. We are all psychologically challenged when we continue to trust governments, industries, doctors, and corporations to have our best interests at heart. Wrong!

For them, we don't exist; we are a shadow, a number, a money supply chain. As pollution gets worse, ask yourself, "How could this happen?" It happens because people don't care about their health now—only when they are sick.

The ideal metaphor for how to view longevity is a see-saw. You are either up with your health and down with disease, or vice versa. Is your health improving or declining at the moment? In addition to discussing the obvious topics like food and fitness, this short book will also include spirituality, meditation, love, happiness, and communal living. Your health is "going down" the see-saw due to stress, glyphosate in your food, tainted water, and polluted air. You're getting "up" with organic food, clean water, outdoor space, rejuvenating exercise, and a fulfilling spiritual life.

Filling your lungs with air during exercise is crucial for supplying your blood with the oxygen it needs to survive. While exercising, the heart rate rises. Increases in breathing rate and depth ensure that more oxygen is taken up by the blood and more carbon dioxide is expelled from it. Every cancer has a trigger, some of which include infections, chemical toxins, or heavy metal poisons. Metabolic alterations that occur early in the course of the cancer's development eventually lead to mutation, which keeps driving genetic changes, growth, and spread. Let's examine how alterations in oxygen metabolism can be one of the earliest metabolic warning indicators of challenging malignancies. Eighth on the periodic table, oxygen plays a crucial function in supplying energy to cells by allowing them to breathe. However, anaerobic, or settings devoid of oxygen, are ideal for malignant, altered cells.

Breathing pure oxygen should be easy: do some regular exercise and live somewhere where there is no pollution. But, millions of people are forced to live and work in polluted cities to make money. The resignation of one's 'holistic' rights in the pursuit of money is questionable. If you want to live a long life then a polluted city is not a good option.

Getting regular exercise and living in a clean environment should make breathing pure oxygen simple. However, millions of people are compelled to live and work in smoggy cities in order to make ends meet. It is problematic to give up one's "holistic" rights for financial gain. A polluted city is not a good choice if you want to live a long life.

According to Nobel Prize winner Dr. Otto Warburg, "the fundamental cause of cancer is the substitution of the respiration of oxygen in normal body cells by a fermentation of sugar," which implies that cancer is brought on by a deficiency of oxygen. Today's modern cancer cell biology has shown he was on the right track as mitochondrial health and shifting to a more oxygen-rich environment may protect healthy cells and further neuter cancer cells.

Exercise, certain foods, and a natural environment are the building blocks (oxygen) for long life. Every page in this book will ask the same question? Are you ready to take in pure oxygen?

Water

Recently, I saw an amazing video by an Indian guru about water. I would like to share his wise words with you here.

Sadguru said: "There are experiments to show water does not respond the same way to every person who approaches it." Over 72 percent of your very physical body is water. If the water does not behave well with you, you are done. Your physical life is going to be a horror story in so many ways. Why wouldn't water respond well to you? To put it in a very simplistic way, if you do not approach this dimension, consciously or unconsciously, appropriately, water may choose not to respond to you well.

So, an enormous amount of systems were established in day-to-day life as to how to treat water. Traditionally, much has been lost, but little remains. People who are conscious of certain things about those who are a little orthodox without knowing why they're doing it are doing the right things. Even today, if you walk into a traditional South Indian home, the water is kept in a certain way. It must be in a metal pot, preferably copper, brass, or some alloy of copper. And, as you will see, they will keep a lamp, and they will have sacred ash smeared on it and a flower on top of it. Of course, many people have shifted to plastic bottles and plastic purifier machines; otherwise, in the night, with a little tamarind and turmeric, the vessel is washed—not with soap—and then water is filled up, and a flower is put on it. And they light a lamp in the night and go to bed. The next morning, they will drink from that. This water is going to behave wonderfully within you. So, I am saying that if you handle water, almost everything that people call "normal life" is generally handled. The agility of the body and the agility of your intelligence largely depend on water. But now you are pumping water through your pipelines from your local waterworks, or whatever you call it. They say if the water is going through, let's say, 50 bends, pumped forcefully, then it drops out of your tap, you take it in your glass, and in terms of molecular structure arrangement, sixty percent of it has turned into poisonous water. But if you hold it in this glass for the next 20 minutes, it will undo itself.

I see in America, people are drinking from a spout like this—straight into their mouths. Many times, when I am thirsty and I am outside, people say, "Sadguru, there's a spout here." I said, "I'll never drink from a spout." In the East, always, the best way to drink water is with your own hands. Not even in a tumbler; you must drink with your own hands. If that's not possible, if somebody gives you water in a metal tumbler, you always hold it with both hands like this. Because it's important that before you drink water, you must touch it, allow that much time, and then drink it; then it behaves differently. And, this may sound like, what to say, some mumbo jumbo story. Well, some people come to their senses only when suffering comes. Some: most people. After things go bad, "Well, you could have told me; I would have loved water." In terms of one's spiritual growth also, water is very important. With what kind of memory and with what kind of attitude are we taking water? I am talking about the memory and attitude of the water. You are responsible for determining how to create that. Your attitude toward the entire thing, not seeing it as a commodity, Water is bigger than your mother, yes, or no? Water is bigger than your God, yes, or no? If you say no, I am going to deprive you of water for the next 24 hours. In 24 hours, you will agree with me. "With the necessary value and the necessary reverence towards it, it has its own way of doing things."

The foundation for a long life is exercise, specific meals, and exposure to nature. The same question will be posed on each page of this book. Ready to breathe in pure oxygen?

The answer to how to stay hydrated with water is typically to drink between 25 percent and 50 percent of your body weight in ounces of water daily. So, if you weigh 160 pounds, you typically want to try to get between 40 and 80 ounces of water a day.

One study, for example, found that American tap water causes rashes and burns on the skin, wears down tooth enamel, and often has arsenic, lead, barium, and other dangerous chemicals in it.

There is also lemon water, celery juice, and hydrogen water to try once you do the research. Hydrogen water is incredibly good too.

Sun

The big three: sun, water, and air They are all around us, so maybe we take them for granted, but we shouldn't. They are the three most important "energies" or "substances" we need to consume every day, and they must be pure; a long life is impossible without showing reverence to these common natural elements. We need water, the best water we can get, to stay alive. We need oxygen coursing through our veins for optimum health, and we need sunlight caressing our skin every day for the energy and the essential vitamin D for health. Because they are natural and free, air, water, and sunlight are extremely beneficial to health.

The authorities were wrong 20 years ago when they said stay out of the sun or you will get skin cancer. This is especially true in 2019, where scientists have discovered that sunblock cremes are absorbed into your blood through your skin within 30 minutes. When you sit in the sun unexposed, without sunscreen, for roughly 10 minutes (between 10 a.m. and 3 p.m.), you likely absorb about 10,000 units of natural vitamin D. Up to 90% of all Westerners are deficient in vitamin D. Vitamin D deficiency is correlated with increased risks of developing common cancers, autoimmune diseases, hypertension, and various infectious diseases. Spending time in the sun without sunscreen is the best way to get vitamin D. When the sun lands on our skin, it converts a substance in our skin to Vitamin D3. You can supplement the sun with fish, eggs, some mushrooms, and raw milk.

Numerous studies have demonstrated that those who are vitamin D deficient are more likely to have health issues and illnesses like cardiovascular disease, metabolic syndrome, several types of cancer, immunological disorders, and unfavorable pregnancy outcomes.

I think we can absorb energy from the sun. With Vitamin D we are getting a boost of energy because we need it to support our immune system. The BBC is exploring the idea that some animals photosynthesize (a chemical reaction that produces sugars) the sun's rays. It is common for science to prove what's true decades after normal people already know it to be true.

Exposure to sunlight increases the brain's release of a hormone called serotonin. Sunlight and darkness trigger the release of hormones in your brain. Exposure to sunlight is thought to increase the brain's release of a hormone called serotonin. Serotonin is associated with boosting mood and helping a person feel calm and focused. At night, darker lighting triggers the brain to make another hormone called melatonin. This hormone is responsible for helping you sleep. Don't be scared of the sun anymore! When more and more doctors are saying, "Go outside and get your daily dose of vitamin D." The scales have tipped back in favor of the sun being good for you and not your enemy. It is crazy when you think about it: governments said, "stay out of the sun or you will get cancer," and now scientists are saying, "stay in the sun or you will get cancer." Common sense prevails.

Exercise

Exercise in daily moderation is essential for a healthy life. For decades, we have been pounded with sports on TV, making it seem like this was the only way to exercise. Now, with large TVs, smartphones, and the internet, any exercise looks pretty good. Seriously, going for a walk, swimming a few laps of the beach, working in your garden, renovating your house, and riding your bike every day will do more for your health than everything else put together. This has been scientifically proven and is the basis for people living for more than 100 years in some areas of the world. So, whatever your age: 5–105, it is imperative you get out of the house and do something, take action, and live forever.

It is wrong thinking—wrong, wrong, wrong—to think, "If I am not working, I need to relax, enjoy, and reward myself after all that horrible work stuff I did (maybe you didn't) today." Everyone, I know, wants to make every minute of their lives special; they don't want to be zombies staring at a screen that makes sounds—many sounds to attract your attention. Maybe you have always been too polite, and you show the same respect to people talking to you on a screen as you do in real life. This is how the advertisers and money lenders want you to react. I often marvel when I see people walk into a shop where a TV is blaring some unfortunate news and look up and listen like they are talking to them personally. I don't have a TV in my home and haven't had one for 12 years. I stopped watching TV one night after realizing I spent more time watching my wife watch TV than I did watching it myself.

In the 1960s, Robin McKenzie, a physical therapist in New Zealand, developed the McKenzie Method. McKenzie believed that "extending the spine could provide significant pain relief to certain patients." Doing so can also help individuals resume their regular daily activities. She has a lot of good things to say about exercise.

We need a transformation that leaves us feeling healthy, energetic, vibrant and well … ageless. We also need to sleep all night. For, without sleep, we don't function. And with all we still have to do in life, we need to function well. That means no more foggy brain, no more sore joints, no more crazy mood swings, and no more weight gain. In fact, we often need to lose at least 15kg of fat that menopause can dump on our bodies.

Yoga, Tai Chi, walking, running, swimming, aerobics, riding a bike, gardening, dancing, and painting the house are easy and fun ways to keep fit. Remember, exercise is the best way you have of feeling younger and longer.

My brother will turn 80 this June. He was a champion football, squash, and tennis player in his 20s. When he retired, he took up bicycle racing and came in second in the world in 2018 in Austria. He says his diet is normal food with no alcohol, smoking, or junk food. He is healthy and very strong, which seems to prove just how good exercise is as we get older. Both my parents played golf every Wednesday and Friday. They didn't get to 100 but were quite fit and strong into their 70s and 80s. Unfortunately, my mother smoked up until the age of 60, which cut her life short in her 70s with a quick onset of emphysema. When my father was in his 50s, he had an accident with refrigeration gas that caused him lung problems when he was in his 80s. They both died of lung problems.

Diet

This book is going to step its way through countless ways to feel younger and longer. Feel free to skip pages and read topics you haven't already read. Pure sunlight, water, and air top the list because they work and because they are, well, essential for life.

Every chapter, though, should be considered equally important because, as Dr. Keith Scott-Mumby from Los Vegas frequently says, "the more you overload your system, the more likely you will get sick, and vice versa." I agree.

There are millions of dollars spent on research on cancer every year, "looking for a cure," when according to Dr. Scott-Mumby, there already is one: don't push your body too far and don't gamble on your health. Make sure your organic food, good sleep, peaceful mind, daily exercise, pure air, water, and sunlight far outweigh your consumption of stress, alcohol, junk food, and mental collapse.

Diet is a big topic and starts with organic food and finishes with chocolate and red wine.

Food is our medicine, and herbs are our medicine too. We should be more aware of this and think more about taking papaya leaf tea for malaria than a pill. Avocados are essential for our health, as are olives (oil) and honey. Garlic is a miracle food, as are broccoli and red onions. Dark chocolate, organic coffee, and natural red wine are also essential to consume daily for optimum health. There are many good websites where you can get all the information you need, in a few weeks, to consciously consume food to remedy your daily ills and problems. Four of the best are draxe.com, naturalnews.com, greenmedinfo.com, and alternative-doctor.com. They are doctors or scientists and can be trusted with accurate or compelling information about diet and health.

I could write 50 pages about diet, but I won't. I want you to start keeping records of what foods, including herbs, leaves, nuts, seeds, vegetables, fruit, oils, grains, juices, mushrooms, seaweeds, and honey, you can eat, first as a cure and then as a prevention for many diseases. These foods are also delicious.

Doctors never ever say, "Food is our medicine," so I condemn them for malpractice and self-interest. They never take the attitude of maximizing all your options for optimum health or survival; I see this as a gross misuse of power and privilege. The only way you can overcome this huge problem is for you to take care of yourself, and if you think you need a doctor, you can communicate with them from a position of power. Here is a small list to get you started; these should be part of your weekly diet (all organic if possible).

Vegetables: broccoli, avocado, all kinds of beans, all kinds of mushrooms, seaweeds, all green vegetables, garlic, red onion, beetroot, pumpkin, and sweet potato.

Oils: olive oil, coconut oil, and avocado oil.

Leaves and seeds: (you can eat much more than you think).

All Fruit in season: jackfruit, mango, pineapple, bananas, and apples.

Grains: oats, sesame seed hulls, flaxseed hulls.

All kinds of nuts: walnuts, cashew, and almond.

Herbs either fresh or dry: ginger, turmeric, astragalus, Andrographis, ashwagandha, holy basil, and CBD oil.

Fluids: pure water, vegetable and fruit juice, lemon water, celery juice, and hydrogen water.

Other wonderful foods: tahini, houmous, dark chocolate, red wine, honey, and coffee. There is a lot more you can add to these lists.

And there are quite a few things not to eat, like alcohol (although natural red wine is good), any processed foods, sodas, sugar, white flour, and rice. Mr. Overton laughs about his "Overton Diet," which includes lots of coffee and whiskey, cigars, butter pecan ice cream, and Campbell's soup. He lived to be 109 years old, so he is clearly saying the Overton Diet is about being happy and feeling good. More about Mr. Overton soon. I agree with him about being happy, BUT! There is a middle path, and that is eating yummy food that is proven to be good for your health, like natural red wine, nuts, mangoes, avocadoes, and dark chocolate. Not many of us have his genes. Ok, Mr. Overton is next.

Richard Arvin Overton

Mr. Overton said: "Yeah I've had a lot of people say God kept you here to help others but I don't know why he kept me here I can't tell you. I ain't talked to Him and He ain't he talked to me.

My name is Richard Arvin Overton I am a hundred and nine years old. I still walk, I still talk and I still drive. I just got my license renewed this year. They give me an eye test. Everything they give me now I pass it. I feel good going on driving. I like to drive myself 'cause other drivers, they drive crazy.

I am the oldest World War II, veteran. I went in the Army in 1940. Made you braver, stronger, I can sleep with every door open here without a lock on it. Ain't scared, no. Ain't nothing gonna bother you. You see a soldier with a gun you don't see him turn around and go back this way. He may go sideways… but he ain't gonna turn around and go back. Don't care how hot them bullets is, he ain't gonna go back. So, when you go in there you just say, well God has got me now. See… He gonna take care of you. If it's your time to go then that bullet is going to get ya. If it ain't your time to go, that bullet's going over your head, it ain't gonna to hit you So, man will kill you but God is the one keep you alive. It wasn't good but we had to go.

I built me a house in 1945 and that's where I have been ever since. It's a nice place to live. Yeah I'm happy with my house. It's all I need. I would buy one thing, I would use that one thing. I wouldn't buy one thing and go buy another and and go buy another. I've got a truck out there and it runs just like I want it, so I just keep it. But I don't fool with a credi card, never. For everything I get I pay cash for it. I got 50 cents a day, that's way back yonder. But I lived out of that. Of course, everything was nickel and dime, three cents. I remember when a man had the first Ford, I was at… Working in the… I think I was picking cotton down there and we heard that he was gonna get a car. We didn't know what a car was, we'd heard about it, but we would never come to town much. My first car was a little old Ford, Model T Ford. Had to get in front and crank it. You remember them, Oh no you wasn't born then, was you? No.... I know you wasn't.

I just sit there and sometimes smoke 12 cigars a day, sometimes more than that. Anybody say "what do you smoke em for?" I just, it just, it makes you feel better. But you can't inhale. Best to go ahead and just blow it out and let it go and forget about swallowing it. If you swallow it, ain't no taste to it; it just makes you cough. I'm doing it the healthy way.

Every time I get up in the morning that cat is sitting there waiting. And either I go to bed sometimes they're sitting there waiting 'cause they wanna get their supper and then they wanna go to bed. But you don't feed a cat too much 'cause he won't eat a rat. I help those cats and they keep me happy. I… I tell the truth they keep me happy, I wanna see my cats every morning.

I wake up at 1 either wake up at 2 or 3… anytime I wake up I just get up. I get me a cup of coffee. Sometimes I drink about four cups of coffee in the morning. This morning I drank about that much whiskey.

I love milk, and fish, corn and soup; I love soup. A lot of people don't like soup and don't drink milk, but I been drinking milk for over… practically all my life. And ice cream. I eat ice cream every night: it makes me happy. I eat butter pecan. If you wanna buy any, you buy butter pecan. And it's the Overton Diet: it's anybody's diet that wanna eat it.

Church is a wonderful place, lovely place. Keeps me goin' makes me feel good. I think that helps me push myself along going to church. You learn something at church too. You learn how to live better; how to treat people. We don't have all the answers, I got to save some of the answers for somebody else to do. And singing, I love that church singing: beautiful. Church is just for everybody. But, you gotta go for one person, that's yourself. Good to have a spiritual life: but you got to live it. It makes …. It makes you feel better.

To have a person around you like MS Love; we get along real nice. Oh, she's 91 years old: you know I'm 109. And yeah, we go to the hospital to see people. We go to the grocery store, we go shopping sometimes. I take her to church, and take her different places, she's just a nice person. Yeah, we have fun together.

I've seen lots and lots of living. But I am still living good; I ain't suffered or nothing. I get what I want. So, I'm still living alright. If you give up you're through! You just doubting yourself. I am, I'm giving you some of my secrets to a long life: if you ever use it. If you don't use it that's your bad luck. My time ain't got here yet. And I don't know when I come here and I don't know when I'm going. You either… neither one of us know when we going.

I may give out but I never give up."

Telomeres

This year's Nobel Prize in Physiology or Medicine is awarded to three scientists who have solved a major problem in biology: how the chromosomes can be copied in a complete way during cell divisions and how they are protected against degradation. The Nobel Laureates have shown that the solution is to be found in the ends of the chromosomes – the telomeres – and in an enzyme that forms them – telomerase.

The telomeres are the caps on the ends of the long, threadlike DNA molecules that make up our chromosomes and carry our genes. It was found by Elizabeth Blackburn and Jack Szostak that the telomeres' distinctive DNA sequence shields the chromosomes from deterioration. The enzyme that creates the telomere DNA, telomerase, was discovered by Carol Greider and Elizabeth Blackburn. These findings clarified how telomeres work and how telomerase constructs them to safeguard the ends of chromosomes.

The long, threadlike DNA molecules that carry our genes are packed into chromosomes, with the telomeres being the caps on their ends. Elizabeth Blackburn and Jack Szostak discovered that a unique DNA sequence in the telomeres protects the chromosomes from degradation. Carol Greider and Elizabeth Blackburn identified telomerase, the enzyme that makes telomere DNA. These discoveries explained how the ends of the chromosomes are protected by the telomeres and that they are built by telomerase.

But where do we find telomerase? That's where the herb Astragalus Membranaceus comes into the picture. Astragalus membraneaceus is a plant native to China. In China, the astragalus roots have been used medicinally for ages, mainly after the roots have aged for four to seven years. Once harvested, the astragalus roots are made into teas, extracts, or tonics. Astragalus is considered a powerful herb that stimulates the immune system and contains powerful antioxidants and flavonoids that contribute to a healthy body and longevity. After years of research, scientists have succeeded in isolating CA-98's Cycloastragalus (CA) molecule from the Astragalus plant.

This is by far the most important thing you can do to live longer. Astragalus root has been known for years as a rejuvenating herb. The herb has been tested for telomerase activity, and it has tested positive. Like all herbs mentioned in this book, if you search for it on the internet, with or without the word "research," you will find everything you need to know. Whether you take it in a more concentrated form depends on how quickly you want to reduce your ageing. I think taking the root as a tonic or tea first is cheaper and will have positive effects. Remember that researching telomeres and telomerase on the internet properly should increase your years on this planet, and it's all scientifically proven.

Flaxseed and Black Sesame Seed Hulls

These simple seeds are a powerhouse of health. A friend of mine started selling a product called Sesamin, which is a concentrated form of black sesame seeds, which are used all over Asia as a powerful herb or supplement. I studied sesame and was shocked to find out how black sesame and flaxseed hulls can improve your health so dramatically, including HIV and cancer. They are both called lignans. Lignans are seriously important for our health and a necessary part of it as well, like CBD oil and the cannabinoid system. When plant lignans are ingested, they can be metabolized by intestinal bacteria to enterolignans, enterodiol, and enterolactone in the intestinal lumen.

Flaxseeds are among the richest sources of plant lignans in the human diet, but they are also good sources of other nutrients and phytochemicals with cardioprotective effects, such as omega-3 fatty acids and fiber.

I have seen proof of Sesamin and properly extracted Flaxseed Lignans curing cancer, liver disease, and arthritis.

Flaxseed is available for free in Africa now to combat HIV.

While many research scientists have understood that inside the flax hull is a treasure chest of anti-cancer lignans, no one has been able to unlock those lignans without destroying them until a Christian farmer in North Dakota named Curtis Rangeloff says that God answered him in response to prayer and showed him how. With the help of his friend Dennis Maw, they figured out how to isolate the hulls with the lignans intact—a process that had previously stumped medical scientists. Previously, removing the soft pulp resulted in its destruction, or more accurately, in destroying much of its medical usefulness. Their proprietary process extracts the lignans in such a way that it provides 1,000 times the cancer cell-destroying capabilities of just plain flax. Both farmers credit learning the secret to this process by attending the World Flax Conference held in Fargo,

ND, for the last 10 years. It was this knowledge, research, and prayers that blessed them with the idea of inventing the world's first chemical-free method of mechanically separating the lignan-rich hulls from the rest of the flax in a manner that prevents rancidity and allows for a stable, effective product for consumer use.

Sesamin is also a lignin that is obtained by a special process. Around 1 kg of black sesame seeds are needed to make 60 Sesamin capsules. Just eating crushed flaxseeds or black sesame seeds won't work. They are certainly healthy, but they don't have the power to cure serious diseases; you need the concentrated versions of these seeds.

Astragalus plus flaxseed or sesame lignans will change your life and are not so expensive.

A Few Herbs

Along with Astragalus, Ginger, Turmeric, Andrographis, Ashwagandha, Garlic, and Ginseng taken every other day, these will dramatically improve your health. This is not a difficult thing to understand. Herbs are amazing and a miracle. If you believe in God, then there is no doubt that you can believe that God created herbs to cure us of all disease. Doctors have stolen this miracle from us because they work for pharmaceutical companies, and they hate herbs because they work better than their products and are way cheaper. Herbs are often used in food, like turmeric and ginger. There is little to fear when you take them. Even doctors and scientists like Dr. Axe and Mike Adams have a lot of information you can read about the efficacy of herbs and how to use them. What you need to fear is your blind faith in doctors. If herbs are from God, where are doctors from?

If you research the internet about common flu viruses, you will discover that doctors have no medicine for them. That's right! There is no cure for viruses like there are antibiotics for bacteria. There are many herbs that can boost your immune system and make it stronger. Andrographis is at the top of this list. Andrographis is used extensively in Germany for the flu. When I have a fever, I mix 1 teaspoon of Andrographis powder with some water and drink it. I feel much better after 30 minutes. Fresh ginger the size of your thumb in a cup of hot water is also helpful. So, doctors have been lying to you for decades when they say go home, drink water, and rest; there is much more you can do.

Turmeric with a pinch of black pepper is the most researched herb in the world at the moment. It can prevent Alzheimer's, reduce inflammation, offer all kinds of pain relief, be good for your digestive system, and much more. Ginseng is a proven tonic. Ashwagandha calms the nervous system and has a host of benefits. All these herbs can be researched on the internet. I highly recommend them, which means I have personal evidence of their power, and I take most of them every week. I like to eat garlic and fresh chilis every day. Dr. Keith Scott-Mumby has articles about sticky blood. I've been taking fresh chilis every day for the past ten years without knowing why. Cayenne pepper and chilis thin your blood. When your blood is thin, it is not sticky like in Dr. Keith's article, so your blood pressure is low to normal and nutrients get to every part of your body where they are needed. Some doctors in America use cayenne pepper to revive heart attack victims.

The most celebrated herbalist in the world is the late Stephen Harrod Buhner. His books are incredible. If you have time and the desire, you will be completely engaged by what he says. No one could be a better herb representative for God's healing herbs than him.

I hope you study herbs and use them every day. There are many sources of information that included safety and doses for adults and children. Put you and your family first and your doctor last: doctors are slowly changing their ways.

The Blue Zones

The Blue Zones are a fantastic resource for learning how to live a long life. Why? because they are home to the greatest number of centenarians in the entire world. They are currently the subject of in-depth research, and the results are straightforward, useful, and simple to apply to every aspect of our life. They engage in daily activities like working on their farms or vegetable gardens, which is why so many of them live to be 100 years old. They love fruits and vegetables like sweet potatoes and don't consume a lot of meat. Every day, they sip a little wine and coffee. They typically have a strong sense of purpose and enjoy living in their communities and families.

Despite regional differences in dietary preferences, Blue Zone diets tend to be plant-based, with up to 95% of daily calories coming from fruits, vegetables, grains, and legumes. Meat and dairy products, as well as sweet foods and drinks, are often avoided by people living in blue zones. Additionally, they avoid eating processed meals.

Foods they typically eat.

Legumes include chickpeas, lentils, black-eyed peas, and pinto beans. Around half a cup a day will strengthen your heart and supply protein, minerals, and vitamins. Plenty of fruit like blueberries, melons, and avocadoes are an important part of their diet as well.

Dark leafy greens like kale, spinach, and Swiss chard supply large quantities of vitamin A and C.

Nuts are packed with protein, minerals, and vitamins. Try to snack on almonds, walnuts, pistachios, cashews, and Brazil nuts every day. Extra virgin olive oil is consumed in large quantities.

Oats and barley are their favorite grains. Like I said earlier, wine, coffee, chocolate, and sweet potatoes are taken often too. There is everything you need on the internet to create a diet and life plan based on these centenarians.

Most of us know how to live like this and how beneficial it is. For people in the Blue Zones, it is a normal cultural practice to do what they are doing. Maybe they have always known this is the secret to a long and happy life. We don't have the same cultural and community support they have, so we need to create our own supportive small communities like our extended families and organize our wonderful future together. The most incredible and fantastic thing about living longer is that it is easy and lots of fun. Let's go. Each chapter of this book reinforces the same thing.

The Mediterranean Diet

This is a famous diet that is quite closely linked to the Blue Zones in Sardinia and Greece. This diet is rich in whole grains, which include wheat, barley, brown rice, buckwheat, oats, bulgur, and quinoa. The whole is the most important part. The whole grain is far superior to processed or white grains.

Fruit is so important that you need to make it around half of what you eat in a day.

Olive oil is without question the pinnacle of the Mediterranean diet. Make sure you buy Extra Virgin.

Fatty fish that is full of Omega 3 fatty acids like herrings, salmon, sardines, mackerel, and tuna

Legumes like beans, peas, and lentils are low in fat and full of protein. Also, chickpeas, kidney beans, and pinto beans are awesome. These are delicious cooked in a stew, soup, or Mexican dish.

Nuts are what you should be eating for a snack at home and at work. Dairy products like kefir and yogurt are delicious and healthy. And wine. Wine is very healthy if it is natural and organic. One glass for women and two for men every day sounds awesome.

This diet is just normal for people in the Mediterranean. It is the same as the Blue Zones in Sardinia and Greece. Dr. Keith Scott-Mumby says there is no such thing as moderation. If you have some soda, junk food, etc. every day, it will eventually bring you down. I think following the Blue Zone lifestyle is the best way to start the next part of your life. Make the change and write down a complete plan about how you will do it. If you just take bits and pieces from everywhere, you will not make the total revolution in health that is needed to live to 100. Make it your new religion. They say it takes 30 days to form a new habit or break an old one. If you don't eat much fruit, now is the time.

With the help of the Blue Zone and Dr. Axe, you have all the tools you and your family need to get started.

Sometimes it is good to buy nuts, olive oil, grains, and legumes in bulk. It is cheaper, and you can buy from a reputable organic food supplier.

Cancer and other diseases are on the rise. Doctors are still using chemotherapy because they will not adopt the obvious cure of "natural foods" because it will put them out of business. Doctors in the US have an enormous conflict of interest when it comes to your health. Just CBD oil alone could reduce their and pharmacy companies' profits by half.

We don't know the future either. Plagues like Ebola and the bird flu can spread quickly. All the foods and medicines in this book will build your immune system and help you fight a plague if it ever comes.

Yoga and Meditation

This book is about natural food, natural medicine, and natural forms of relaxation and exercise. Again, doctors and industry say "natural" is some kooky, hippie thing. This could not be further from the truth. Nature is perfect. What humanity makes is not. cigarettes, alcohol, TV dinners, big macs, automobiles, robots, Wi-Fi, polluted cities, corrupt politicians, oligarchs, wars, inequality, poverty, pharmaceuticals, fractured relationships, factory farms, glyphosate, computer games, education, drugs, sexual promiscuity, TV, movies, and all junk food. Humans cannot improve on nature, and they never will. All they do is profit from it. If you think carefully about your life, you will concede that it is love, health, and happiness that are important, not all the expensive junk people make for profit with no regard for your wellbeing in any way. So, change how you think about the word "natural" (if you haven't already) and give thanks to God for this bounty of beauty and perfection. Our God must come first and always be at the pinnacle of common sense and truth, not man.

With this in mind, yoga, tai chi, and meditation are natural forms of exercise and relaxation that you can do for free once you are accomplished with their techniques. They are soul-restoring, de-stressing, and centered activities that holistically improve every aspect of your life. Unfortunately, books like the Bible and the Koran don't stress these kinds of activities, as they were written a long, long time ago, when people were quite ferocious. If you are seriously wanting to improve your health and live to 100 (I doubt you can), you will need some form of peaceful and relaxing exercise or activity. Gardening, walking, swimming, yoga, tai chi, meditation, painting, dancing, and reading are all beneficial to a long life. The more, the merrier. Our mind is quite negative when we contemplate new activities in our lives, often saying things like "I have no time or money." This is where a giant leap of faith comes in. No matter what you want to do in your life—tell your husband you love him; change your job; travel; lose weight; give up alcohol and cigarettes—you will always need a leap of faith to bypass your negative mind. If you don't know already, your mind is always trying to keep you in some kind of confinement based on your childhood and past experiences. It is quite simple: don't ever listen to your mind, and if you do, recognize just how negative and punishing it is. Don't think! Feel it and do it.

One good book on this subject is "Outwitting the Devil" by Napoleon Hill. This book certainly changed my life. It is hard to recognize how destructive our minds can be without some help from someone who has control over them. One good example is meditation. Normally, I can't sit still for more than five minutes. My mind is hyperactive. Then, one day, I realized the truth. My mind is preventing me from meditating by simply saying things like, "Your back hurts. You can't meditate." Now I can tell it to stop, whether I am trying to meditate or not. Yay! This is a life-changer.

Fasting and Detox

When I was 30, I had my first coffee enema. I bought a red rubber bulb with a tube and some coffee. I made a warm cup of coffee and had a good friend suck it up into the bulb and then insert it into my rectum. I was lying down on my side. They slowly squeezed the coffee up into my intestines. Around 30 minutes later, it all came whooshing back out, full of different colored powders and all sorts of weird things. I could not believe my eyes. The enema worked; I had gotten rid of all sorts of chemicals out of my body. These days, if I want to detox my insides, I eat a few bowls of fruit and drink three or four bottles of water. After an hour or two, it comes whooshing through me and cleans me out. This is one really good way to detox, even if you only do it once in a lifetime.

There are other ways to detox, like drinking juices. Celery juice is very popular. You juice one whole organic celery and drink it first thing after waking up. You will find tons of information on celery juicing on the internet. Some say it changed their lives, while others say it was good at first but they stopped doing it after a few weeks to save money and maybe because they felt clean enough on the inside.

Even if you've never drank anything green in your life, it's likely that you've heard of celery juice. Because suddenly it looks like everyone is drinking it. They not only consume it, but they also vouch for it. Anthony William, a medical psychic, has been juicing (and talking about) celery for years, so it's nothing new for him. William explains why he thinks it's a magic elixir and how he takes it.

Drinking lemon water first thing in the morning is also a popular way to detox. The liver is extremely active during sleep since this is the body's time to restore and regenerate. Drinking enough water, especially in the morning, helps make sure that the body can perform these jobs most effectively. There is even some evidence that lemon juice can help stimulate proper stomach acid and bile production. Lemon water helps with better skin, helps you lose a little bit of weight, and aids digestion. It is important to drink a few glasses of water in the morning when you wake up; adding lemon juice makes it even better.

It is a great plant to use moringa. You can purchase the powder made from the leaves of the moringa tree and combine it with juice or water. A small tree from India, Pakistan, and Nepal known as Moringa oleifera, also called the horseradish tree, ben tree, or drumstick tree, has been used for centuries in Eastern countries to treat and prevent illnesses like diabetes, heart disease, anemia, arthritis, liver disease, and respiratory, skin, and digestive disorders. Vitamins, minerals, and amino acids are abundant in moringa. It has considerable levels of calcium, potassium, protein, and vitamins A, C, and E. It combats inflammation and free radicals. Blood sugar levels are decreased. Your heart will thank you for it. It enhances mental performance while safeguarding the liver. It fights against both germs and fungus. You can make a tea out of moringa or add it to your smoothie. In human testing, the leaf powder was pronounced safe, even in higher dosages than usual. The powder has a delicate flavor and produces a light, somewhat earthy moringa tea.

State of Mind

How we think and feel, what motivates us and what we are striving to achieve will affect our health. I like to follow the Buddhist and Christian path. Helping others is high on that list. What goes around comes around. You don't need to be a genius to understand that we all need to help each other. Helping others is our biggest challenge because we spend most of our time thinking we need the most help.

When my daughter was born, it really helped to take my mind off all my problems and focus on taking care of her. This same formula has helped ever since: the more I help others, the better I feel because I am not thinking about myself so much. Also, this is the most basic ingredient in the big cake of life. We are not beings in isolation; we are all connected and part of a big galactic team.

I have read a few times that a God works through people; people are the messengers of a God, and this is how it all works. I am pretty sure if you don't understand this simple reality, you will have a sad life because "no one loves me." Like I said earlier, when my daughter was born, a lot of this crazy emotional baggage fell away and I could see better. One step further in this idea makes you like an angel. The more you do God's bidding, the more God will bid you, with the accompanying rewards. Wow, say that again. If we do God's work, become part of the team, and help others, we will be rewarded with a happy life and a long one.

It is also important to speak your truth to your family and friends and do the things you always wanted to do but never found the time to do. Don't be too serious; learn to forgive and forget; and follow some of your dreams. If you follow the ideas in this book, you will live long enough to have a giant bucket list. We all have two lives: the cultural one and the soul one. They should be kept in balance. No matter how many bills and problems based on survival we have, we must never forget the dreams of our soul and why we are here. Making a living, getting married, and bringing up children Buying a home and a car These are the cultural things we all do, but the soul wants to be a painter or write books. The soul wants to meditate and find a spiritual path, travel the world, and find a cure for cancer. If you work hard all your life for your children, remember, they will take whatever you give them.

There is no better time than now to follow your dreams, set your soul free, and do what you came here to do. Nothing else can make you feel younger or older, depending on your actions.

Sleep

There is a lot of research these days that says we need a minimum of eight hours of sleep. I have some friends who like to get up at 4 a.m. so they can do more. They seem a little crazy to me. Sleep is an easy thing to do, yet it is the healthiest thing as well. A good night's sleep restores body and soul. If you have trouble sleeping, you should do everything you can to fix the problem.

The best herbs for a good night's sleep are valerian, chamomile, lemon balm, passionflower, lavender, and peppermint. You can buy them separately and brew a wonderful good night's cup of tea, or buy them already mixed.

Exercise is always a good way to get a good night's sleep too. Swimming, riding a bike, going for an evening run, or dancing to dawn

"If a problem is fixable, if a situation is such that you can do something about it, then there is no need to worry." If it's not fixable, then there is no use in worrying. "There is no benefit in worrying whatsoever." The Dalai Lama

A Bucket List

Watch the movie and then make your own. This a great way to organize your dreams.

An Australian nurse several years working with patients who had less than three months to live, recorded their thoughts, and regrets.

Here are the five biggest regrets of the dying:

1) I wish I'd had the courage to live a life true to myself, not the one others expected of me.

This was the most common regret of all the people lying on their deathbeds. When they realized that life was over, they had the ability to look back with clarity. Unfortunately, many of these people saw a life with dreams left unfulfilled.

Most people had not honored even half of their dreams and had to die, knowing that it was due to choices they had made or not made.

2) I wish I hadn't worked so hard

Every single male patient had this regret. The men said they missed so much of their relationships and friendships because they simply worked too hard. While women spoke of this regret, the majority were from a different generation that had not been the breadwinners.

Don't spend so much time at work that you forget to live your life. Find a work-life balance so you can earn money, work on your passion, and still have plenty of time to create beautiful relationships.

3) I wish I had the courage to express my feelings

Many people suppressed their feelings in order to keep peace with others. As a result, they settled for a mediocre existence and never became who they were truly capable of becoming.

Don't be afraid to express your true feelings, good or bad. Holding in resentment, bitterness, and anger is toxic for your soul. Express yourself, deal with the situation, and move on. Don't hold on to negative emotions any longer than you need to.

4) I wish I had stayed in touch with my friends

Often, they would not truly realize the full benefits of old friends until their dying weeks, and it was not always possible to track them down. Many had become so caught up in their own lives that they had let golden friendships slip over the years.

Frequently, they would not fully appreciate the benefits of long-time friends until the latter weeks of their lives, and it was not always easy to locate them. Many people have allowed cherished friendships to lapse over the years due to becoming mired in their own lives.

5) I wish I had let myself be happier

Many people did not understand that choosing happiness until it was too late. They had continued to act in the same patterns and routines. Their emotions and daily lives both overflowed with the alleged "comfort" of familiarity.

Always keep in mind that you have the power to choose happiness. Decide to be joyful. Decide to be lively, alive, and upbeat. On their deathbed, no one ever complained that their life had been too happy.

Change the way you live your life by applying these lessons from "Five Regrets of the Dying". Choose to be joyful as often as you can, spend time with the people you love, and share your emotions. You have the option to live a better life every day; the decision is yours!

Outwitting the Devil

If we spend most of our days and nights fighting the devil, we will surely die young. For me, the devil is all the negative thoughts that can go around in your head and then venture outwards into the world of reality. We are part animal and part angel. When our animal overpowers us, we seek to fulfill its desires for sex, money, and power. There are so many examples of this in my own life I am embarrassed to admit. But I will use one of a friend of mine who developed a "fantasy desire" for his best friend's wife. His desires grew and grew until he "lost sight of himself" the devil in his mind had taken full control. He started to stalk her, hiding in bushes, dreaming about their life together (she had no idea, and was not interested if she did) He finally admitted his love for this woman to his wife, she left him, he was alone, he went even crazier and finally killed himself. This is the real devil and he has the power to send you to a hell of your own making. But the devil is not a separate entity it is the animal nature of all humans that can break free of logic and all sanity: and grow out of control in our mind.

My favorite book of all time is called "Outwitting the Devil" by Napoleon Hill. This book is the key to every door we need to open. Bestselling author Napoleon Hill reveals the seven principles of good that allow us to triumph over obstacles…and find success.

Using his legendary ability to get to the root of human potential, Napoleon Hill digs deep to reveal how fear, procrastination, anger, and jealousy prevent us from realizing our personal goals. This long-suppressed parable, once considered too controversial to publish, was written by Hill in 1938 following the publication of his classic bestseller, Think and Grow Rich. Annotated and edited for a contemporary audience by Rich Dad, Poor Dad and Three Feet from Gold co-author Sharon Lechter, this book is profound, powerful, resonant, and rich with insight.

Monsanto and Glyphosate

We can see wars on TV. We know about poisons that can kill us instantly. We used to trust our politicians... We can make the decision to buy organic food, exercise, and sleep all night, but we can't test our food for glyphosate.

The Health Ranger, Mike Adams, can find it and has found that most processed foods are saturated with it. Why? Because Monsanto sells it as an herbicide to all American farmers to kill weeds. There is only one problem: it is banned nearly everywhere in the world because it causes cancer. Yes, corporations have so much power in the U.S. that they can pay off politicians to support their continued use, even though it kills. The main reason people go "organic" is because of glyphosate. We cannot live long lives when companies like Monsanto keep poisoning us. You should do your own research into glyphosate and decide if this alone is the reason you must buy organic food for you and your family.

Jurors award $289 million to a man they say got cancer from Monsanto's Roundup weedkiller. The potential carcinogenic properties of glyphosate are the subject of widespread scientific debate. The US Environmental Protection Agency said in a 2017 draft risk assessment that the herbicide "is not likely to be carcinogenic to humans," while the European Food Safety Authority maintains a similar stance. Bayer, which acquired Monsanto in 2018, said the same year that glyphosate is a "safe and efficient weed control tool."

In 2015, however, the World Health Organization's International Agency for Research on Cancer classified glyphosate as "probably carcinogenic to humans." Moreover, the chemical has triggered multiple lawsuits from people who believe that exposure to the herbicide caused their non-Hodgkin's lymphoma. In 2017, more than 800 people were suing Monsanto; by the following year, that figure was in the thousands.

Roundup (glyphosate) is now owned by Bayer, and they continue to promote it around the world. This example of corporate influence over the government is horrific. We elect people to govern for us, the people, but what they do is govern for corporations. This creates a vicious profit cycle. Consumers buy processed food, consume poisons, go to the doctor with cancer, and die in the hospital with cancer. The corporations get rich by making you sick, then curing you of the very disease they gave you, usually resulting in death and a loss of huge amounts of money.

A God

A controversial topic

When I say "god," I mean the Red Indian God, the Hindu, Muslim, and Buddhist God. The Aboriginal and Māori God The Christian and Jewish Gods and all the others from the beginning of time I think most people recognize the wonder of creation. We, as societies all around the planet, create beliefs, rituals, and books to connect with greater powers than ourselves. In each society, children are "exposed" to these cultural beliefs and often accept them as true; thus, they become part of a collective of worshippers and believers. But there are a couple of problems with this system. The first one is a book. For example, the Bible is touted as the word of God, which it isn't; it was written by people like you and me. And the second is the lack of understanding that" whatever created us and the universe" did it (and continues to do it) regardless of what we call them.

Spiritual life is essential: for a long one. To have an open mind and accept all people's beliefs as different strands of hair on God's head is a way to learn more and live longer. There have been millions killed in the name of God. When the English Christians went to America, Canada, Australia, and New Zealand, they wiped out millions of the indigenous people who owned the land—land that was essentially stolen by Christians. To be a Christian, Muslim, or Hindu is to be something created by humans, not a God. The only way to know a god is to understand your own true nature. An open and inquiring mind will help you prosper and blossom, leading to inner peace, happiness, and a long life.

Is having faith in God the key to happiness? A new study seems to suggest so, having found that the happiest people in any society or culture tend to be those with strong religious convictions who actively engage with others in regular community worship.

The Pew Research Center looked at data from the United States and more than two other countries, uncovering that "actively religious" folks, meaning those who go to church on a regular basis, are more likely to self-identify as "very happy" than folks who are "inactively religious" or "religiously unaffiliated."

Natural Medicine Practitioners

Naturopaths, homoeopaths, chiropractors, masseurs, acupuncturists, Chinese herbalists, Reiki practitioners, yoga teachers, and meditation teachers belong to the natural medicine and healthy lifestyle group, versus doctors.

When we take responsibility for our own health, we must do four things. Firstly, find a good doctor. Secondly, find a good natural healer. Thirdly, create your own health bible, and fourthly, make a health plan for diet, exercise, supplements, and spiritual wellbeing and stick to it. Do it.

Health has gotten much more complicated because we now have access to so much information on the internet, so we have more options. There are thousands of people these days who go to see their doctor and end up telling the doctor what he should do. If doctors don't change, then we won't need them in another 10 years because we will all be better at the issue of health than them. Yes, I am pretty anti-doctors, anti-Catholic, anti-government, and anti-schools. Why? because they don't have our best interests at heart. Doctors show little concern for actual health. The Pope has a secret library of knowledge, governments hold all the power, and schools are systems that need their own management team for their survival.

When left alone, humans can do a good job of taking care of themselves. We can take care of our health, our wisdom, our own governance, and our relationships. I often wonder why we have governments. What do they really do? Whatever it is, it's expensive, and we are paying.

Natural healers are a good option for extra advice and diagnosis of our health, as is this book.

CBD Oil

CBD oil is the biggest breakthrough in health "ever." It is a powerhouse cure for disease and also an amazing preventative. Scientists now agree that we have a cannabinoid system that is part of our physiology. The most powerful cannabinoid is CBD oil (it's legal).

CBD oil is now mainstream in America and hopefully coming soon to the rest of the world. There is a lot of information on the internet about CBD oil, and I cannot recommend it highly enough for virtually all diseases, including cancer. This really is a revolution in health care and has been a long time coming. Here is a link to Dr. Axe and his helpful information about CBD oil. https://draxe.com/cbd-oil-benefits/ CBD is one of 60 compounds derived from the cannabis plant. It is the major non-euphorigenic component of Cannabis sativa and belongs to a class of ingredients called cannabinoids. Our body has a system called the cannabinoid system, which needs cannabinoids to function. CBD is the most powerful form of cannabinoids and should be the very first thing you try if you are suffering from any degenerative diseases like cancer or Parkinson's. Stress, nausea, neurological disorders, diabetes, heart problems, leaky gut, and skin diseases all greatly benefit from CBD oil.

Other, but less powerful forms of Cannabinoids which are: essential oils of rosemary, black pepper, ylang-ylang, lavender, cinnamon, and cloves. Echinacea, truffles, cacao, helichrysum, omega-3 fats, kava, maca, copaiba, and holy basil.

Summary

In the past five years, we have been given proof by scientists about how to extend our lives. This gives us the tools and knowledge to live to 100 years, if we so desire. I want to live to 100 just because I can; it's normal and possible if we follow their findings. In the Blue Zones, they eat simple, healthy foods that include olive oil, legumes, vegetables, and fruit. They do moderate exercise every day, spend time with friends and family, and enjoy a glass of wine. Since scientists discovered telomeres and telomerase, other scientists have discovered what supplements will lengthen your life, like astragalus. Just telomerase and the Blue Zone lifestyle are more than enough to extend your life and make you stronger and happier for longer. So, it's a good idea to adopt these two amazing protocols first.

If you want to make sure you are doing your best, then the rest of the topics in this book (including making your life have a purpose) will provide extra support. Now is the best time to start this journey, never mind your age. Now is better than when you become sick. This book is primarily about prevention. Take your power back, manage your own health and happiness, and do it now. Because once you are sick, you will feel powerless and succumb to the rigors of conservative medicine and hospitals that have their own interests before yours. I have seen it time and again with friends and family, and to be honest, I will fight to the end with my bags of herbs and bottles of reverse osmosis water.

Recent information that has come to light indicates that the best way to stay young is to skip a meal every other day or fast one day a week. Also, take 1 teaspoon of resveratrol. Have an icy cold bath sometimes. Don't overeat, ever. Take Metformin and AMPK; they are good; and either take hydrogen tablets or inhale hydrogen 3 times a week. This information comes from years of research.

Many thanks for purchasing this book

roditch@protonmail.com

www.ingramcontent.com/pod-product-compliance
Lightning Source LLC
Chambersburg PA
CBHW051404280526
45784CB00007B/3086